95 Surprisingly Effective Natural Ways To Fight Acne

Try these popular, proven effective natural ways to enjoy the clear, radiant skin you deserve... starting now.

By Calvert Gamwell

Edited by Amber Henry

Table of Contents

Introduction 4

Top 95 Natural Ways To Fight Acne 5
  Diet and Lifestyle..5
  Vitamin and Mineral Supplements 22
  Essential Herbs, Amino Acids and Antioxidants...........29
  Other Natural Remedies and Topical Treatments 37

Frequently Asked Questions.......................59
  1. What is acne?...59
  2. What causes acne?....................................59
  3. What are the types of acne? 65
  4. How many people have acne? 67
  5. What is the impact of acne? 68
  6. Is there a cure for acne? 68
  7. Will my acne go away naturally?...............69
  8. Should I take prescription drugs for acne? 69

Introduction

Okay. So you've got acne.

You've tried everything. But it still won't go away.
The first thing to tell yourself is that you are not alone: Studies show over 60 million Americans have acne, including three out of four teenagers. This makes acne the most common medical condition in the United States.

The second thing to remember is that millions of people have tried thousands of different acne remedies over the years.

The good news is: now you can benefit from their experiments and experiences to find the best natural acne-fighting remedies for you... without spending a lot of money on expensive over-the-counter products or suffering from the side effects commonly seen with prescription drugs.

So, if you have acne, take heart. You have the power to make your acne go away for good.

With the right attitude, diet, and lifestyle – combined with the right natural remedies – you can look and feel like the person you want to be... bright, bold and blemish-free.
Here's how to get started today!

Top 95 Natural Ways To Fight Acne

From grandma's honey and oatmeal facials to the latest medical and scientific findings, this book is dedicated to helping you get beyond the hype and get into the healing.

Carefully researched and compiled with safe, simple, and surprisingly effective natural ways to fight acne – many of the tips covered in this book have been included due to the number of positive reviews they have received from acne sufferers over the years. Each remedy has also been included based upon its non-invasive and non-toxic natural properties, availability, low cost and ease of use.

Take advantage of these powerful, practical and proven effective ways to reduce the frequency, severity and longevity of your breakouts; learn everything you need to know about acne, antibiotics and more in the Frequently Asked Questions section; and get the answers you need to become acne-free for life!

Diet and Lifestyle

#1: Drink water throughout the day.

You've heard it a thousand times. Drink lots of water, especially if you have acne. Experts recommend that you drink at least half of your body weight in ounces of water per day. The best way to make this happen is to carry around a measured quart or liter bottle of H2O and sip from it regularly during your day.

So if you weigh 120 pounds (54.4 kilograms), you need to drink at least 60 ounces or two liters of water per day.

This equates to slightly less than eight 8-oz glasses of water, which is also roughly equivalent to three pints, a quart and a half or 1.7 liters.

Proper hydration pays off in a myriad of acne-fighting ways from preventing redness and dryness to maintaining smoother, healthier-looking skin. It also helps you experience a more efficient digestive system, improved energy and weight loss to a speedier detoxification process, which helps the body flush acne toxins faster. This helps you control existing breakouts and prevent new ones from forming. So drink up on a daily basis to keep your acne at bay.

#2: Get plenty of rest: at least 7 – 9 hours per night.

You've heard the term "get your beauty rest." Well, guess what? – It really works, particularly when you have acne.

Getting enough rest actually does far more for your skin than a whole shopping cart full of beauty creams and acne medications. When you get the right amount of rest, your skin will actually look clearer, smoother, less inflamed and more radiant and refreshed. Here's how it works.

First, as you sleep, your skin rejuvenates itself. The daily cycle of your old, dead skin calls being replaced with fresh new skin cells occurs faster while you sleep.

Second, your skin has to fight off the sun's harmful UV rays and other environmental pollutants everyday, which can also lead to acne and other skin conditions. Your skin actually repairs itself from this daily damage while you sleep.

Third, getting enough sleep can actually help prevent acne by helping correct any hormonal imbalances that are occurring in your body. Remember that hormonal imbalances cause too much sebum to be produced. Sebum is the oily liquid that clogs your pores and causes acne. When you sleep, your brain regulates and balances your body's hormones, including androgens. As a result, your sebum production becomes more stabilized to help keep your skin more blemish-free.

Finally, sleep helps you succeed in all of your other acne-fighting endeavors as well. Studies show people who get adequate rest are able to focus and concentrate better, think more clearly and positively, have stronger willpower, make healthier food and lifestyle choices, exercise more often, enjoy stronger immune systems and cope more successfully with stress.

So get your rest to look and feel your best.

Average sleep requirements per day.

Age	Hours of Sleep
1-3 years old	12-14 hours
3 -5 years old	11-13 hours
5-12 years old	10-11 hours
13-19 years old	9-10 hours
Young Adult	7-9 hours
Middle Age	7-9 hours
Senior	7-9 hours

Source: National Sleep Foundation

#3: Eat lots of fruits and vegetables.

Your food choices have an enormous impact on your life, not to mention your acne. Research shows that eating a healthy diet – which includes seven to nine servings of fruits and vegetables per day – can have a remarkably positive effect on your skin health, immune and digestive system, energy level, and ability to concentrate and handle problems more productively. Fresh fruit and leafy green vegetables also contain more water and nutrients in them than other foods, which helps bring about a marked improvement in the quality of your complexion.

A healthy diet also includes lean proteins like almonds, chicken, turkey, fish and legumes and healthy fats like olive oil. It does not include sugary, starchy or carbohydrate-rich foods, which can aggravate your acne.
So, instead of feasting on fast food or snacking on cookies, candies and chips – try a fresh salad, carrot sticks, or an apple instead.

#4: Avoid sugary and greasy foods.

Diets high in sugar and carbohydrates such as donuts, rich desserts and deep fried foods have been associated with acne, as well as with a higher level of yeast in the body. More yeast can lead to a variety of discomforting conditions from infections to fatigue, not to mention those bothersome oily bumps.

#5: Address your possible food allergies.

Many acne cases, as well as other skin conditions such as eczema, have been found to be associated with food allergies.

When you consume a food that you are allergic to, continuous toxic reactions take place in your body, releasing a high degree of toxins. This leads to inflammation in the skin resulting in clogged pores, thereby causing acne.

Keep in mind that consuming one or more of the following food groups can be causing or aggravating your acne. Try avoiding one or more of these foods or food groups listed below on an experimental basis to see if your acne condition improves.

#6: Steer away from red meat.

According to information posted on science2day.info, as well as other sources, red meat is known to trigger acne.

Animal proteins are difficult to digest as compared to the vegetable ones. The waste products left in the body may be released through the skin, and this can result in acne. Moreover, there are a lot of hormones fed to livestock these days. This means consuming red meat can lead to a rise in your hormone levels, which may result in pimples.

#7: Beware of dairy products.

Dairy products also may have a negative impact on the skin. In the past several years, numerous studies have emerged concluding that the link between milk and acne is strong, with one study even finding a 44% higher incidence of severe acne among those who drink two or more glasses of milk per day.

This particular study, conducted in 2005, found the strongest association for skim milk intake, suggesting that fat content was not a contributing factor, but rather the hormones and other allergenic proteins found in milk. So why is it that one of nature's most seemingly perfect foods can wreak such havoc on our skin?

Milk increases sebum (oil) production: Almost all commercially available milk comes from pregnant cows. Milk from pregnant cows contains DHT (dihydrotestosterone) precursors, which signal the skin glands to increase sebum production.

Milk contains an array of powerful growth hormones: One of the most potent hormones found in milk is called Insulin-Like Growth Factor-1 (IGF-1). This hormone not only increases sebum production, it also stimulates the growth of new skin cells.

The faster new skin cells grow, the faster they die, leaving more cells behind on the skin to clog pores.

Drinking milk significantly increases insulin levels: Higher insulin levels are associated with increased sebum production, as well as higher levels of IGF-1 and sex hormones in the body. All of these hormones have been conclusively linked to acne.

Milk increases inflammation: The allergenic proteins found in milk stimulate the body's immune system to attack, causing inflammation. As a result, blocked pores can turn into large and painful blemishes.

In conclusion, if you think milk may be contributing to your acne, you might try cutting back or eliminating milk completely from your diet for a few months to see if this makes a difference.

#8: Evaluate your egg eating habits.

Eggs are considered another possible food allergen that can trigger acne. Generally it is the egg yolk that is believed to be the cause. If you are an egg lover with acne, try switching to egg whites.

#9: Pass on the processed foods.

Processed foods contain quite a few preservatives and additives made with toxins that may trigger acne breakouts. Refined sugar or artificial sweeteners can also be behind breakouts for those with acne prone skin. Processed foods that may affect your acne include:

- Sugary breakfast cereals.
- Canned foods with high sodium or fat.
- Breads and pastas made with refined white flour.
- High-calorie snacks like chips and candies.
- Frozen foods and dinners loaded with sodium.
- Packaged breads, cakes and cookies.
- Boxed meal mixes high in fat and sodium.
- Processed meats like hot dogs, bologna and ham.

#10: Stay away from wheat, gluten and grains.

Many foods, including the processed ones, contain wheat, gluten and grains and these ingredients have also been shown to cause or aggravate acne.

This is because these kinds of foods are quickly converted into sugars by your body; and these sugars are what acne-causing bacteria and parasites feed on.

So try reducing your intake of calories from certain high-carb, high-glycemic-index foods made with wheat and grains like biscuits, bread, and pasta. This may alleviate your breakouts. You may also want to try going gluten-free for awhile to see if this helps.

#11: Cut back on caffeine.

Caffeine containing foods and drinks like chocolates, coffee, tea and other cola drinks are also known to be among the most common foods that cause acne. Caffeine stimulates the adrenalin glands to release stress hormones, which increase your stress and lead to acne. Caffeine also disturbs your deep sleep cycle. Since this is the time your body needs each day to regulate hormones, physically repair itself and detox – any disturbance in your sleep can cause your health to decline and your acne to get worse.

#12: If you drink alcohol, only drink in moderation.

Moderation is defined as one or two drinks per day, at the most. Beyond that, alcohol is bad for your skin and your acne. It has a dehydrating effect on the body, damages the liver (reducing its ability to remove toxins from the body) and drains moisture from your skin. This adversely affects your acne and can make your skin more wrinkle-prone over the long run.

Heavy alcohol use over time also dilates the blood vessels and capillaries in the skin, giving the face a redness or flush that will not go away. Alcohol also robs the body of vitamin A, an important antioxidant in skin-cell regeneration.

#13: Don't smoke.

This is a no-brainer. Nicotine reduces blood and oxygen

flow to the skin, robbing it of the nutrients needed to fight and heal acne. This reduced nutrient flow also steals the skin's normal glow and leaves it with a duller, more greyish tone. Smoking also destroys the skin's natural elasticity and promotes wrinkles. Smoking is also known to be toxic and carcinogenic for the rest of the body as well.

#14: Cleanse and moisturize your skin twice per day.

Maintain excellent personal hygiene habits. Keep your skin clean, washed and as sweat-free as possible when you're not exercising.

The build-up of dirt and oil in the skin is another major cause of acne, along with the daily accumulation of dead skin. Experts advise gently washing your face and other acne areas twice per day with a mild, natural, non-drying soap, as well as after sweating and exercising.

Remove all make-up and dirt at night before bed. Avoid antibacterial soaps as they can be too harsh for your face. Don't scrub or wash your face repeatedly, as this will only irritate or exacerbate your condition.

If you have oily or sensitive skin, wash your face and body with a dye- and fragrance-free cleanser. Remember to keep acne prone skin well hydrated and moisturized as dry skin can sometimes aggravate acne.

Follow the skincare regimen of cleansing, toning and moisturizing everyday and do not forget to exfoliate your skin once a week, if this is appropriate for your skin type.

If you follow this skincare regimen, it will keep oil, dirt, bacteria and other debris from building up in your pores, thus helping to prevent or lessen the severity of your breakouts.

#15: Try washing without soap.

Although you may be using a gentle natural soap to wash your acne areas, your cleanser may in fact be contributing to your breakouts. Try washing with warm water only, or using raw or Manuka honey to cleanse and see if this doesn't reduce the frequency or severity of your blemishes.

#16: Use only non-comedogenic cosmetics.

Greasy or oily skin creams and cosmetics can also clog your pores, especially if you already have oily skin. Use only cosmetics that read non-comedogenic on the label as they do not increase the skin's level of oil.

#17: Don't squeeze or pop your pimples.

The tendency to pick or pop your pimples is almost irresistible. Try to avoid it, as popping pimples can push infected material further into the skin, leading to more swelling and redness, and even scarring. If you must pop them, try using a comedone extractor instead. Also, be sure to sanitize the area with rubbing alcohol before and after the extraction to prevent reinfection.

#18: Comb or pull your hair back.

Hair contains oils and collects dirt and other particles that can contribute to your acne. If you have acne, comb or tie your hair away from your face. Also, shampoo daily with an organic or natural shampoo.

#19: Wash your sheets and pillowcases once a week.

Dirt, oil and bacteria can build up on your sheets after a very short time. You also shed millions of skin cells each night as part of the body's natural skin regeneration process. Clean sheets are not only more hygienic, they're more comfortable too.

#20: Wear sunscreen.

Daily sunscreen use is especially important if you are using acne medications. Many of the anti-acne drugs and topical creams on the market today cause the skin to be more vulnerable to UV radiation – putting you at increased risk for severe sunburn, skin damage, premature aging, and skin cancer.

Plus, although a tan may help temporarily camouflage breakouts and discoloration caused by acne, some studies have shown that lying in a tanning bed or out in the sun may actually cause increased oil production, thus increasing the incidence of acne. So, if you're out in the sun, limit your exposure to 20–30 minutes per day and wear sunscreen.

#21: Get regular exercise.

Physical exercise energizes all of your body's organs to go on the attack against acne. As you exert yourself, sweat pours out through your pores. This enables your body's largest organ, your skin, to eliminate toxins and flush out millions of other acne-causing bacteria and debris from deep within your cells.

At the same time, your heart and lungs are pumping more blood and oxygen into your system, sending additional nutrients to your skin and other organs. This improves your skin's cell regeneration and collagen production. It also helps the skin battle back against pollution and other environmental toxins.

This extra blood and oxygen flow also helps slow excess sebum oil production. It also helps soften impacted areas and heal clogged pores; and this in turn lessens inflammation and redness while also giving the rest of your skin a healthier glow.

Your kidneys, pancreas and liver put this added nutrient flow to work by more actively processing foods, stabilizing enzymes and eliminating toxins and other acne-producing impurities from the body.

Meanwhile, with the increased blood and oxygen flow to your brain, it can do a better job of regulating and stabilizing your acne-causing hormonal imbalances. Even better, the brain produces mood-enhancing endorphins that calm and reduce anxiety and stress, eliminating the future outbreaks these conditions can create.

Regular exercise also improves your metabolic rate and digestive process to help you maintain a healthy weight. Getting your body pumping enables your brain to focus, concentrate, think and plan more clearly. And, it helps you sleep better giving you the energy and willpower to make healthier food and lifestyle choices – further minimizing the incidence and severity of your outbreaks. Finally, the acne-fighting benefits of exercise often last for several days after your workout session is done.

So try to exercise for 30 minutes or more at least three times per week. Be sure to hydrate before, during and after.

#22: Reduce your stress.

It's practically impossible to live a completely stress-free life in today's wired and wireless world. On top of that, having acne causes stress, which in turn causes more acne because stress increases sebum oil production further clogging your pores. It's a vicious cycle you need to work on breaking each and every day.

Start with the basics. Get enough rest. Drink plenty of water and eat a healthy diet. Make a list of what you need and want to accomplish each day.

Stay focused, organized and proactive. Tackle the tough jobs and assignments first. Don't procrastinate and let problems, issues, chores and other responsibilities build up on you, as this leads to even more stress.

Exercise, yoga and deep breathing also enable you to keep your stress in check. You might also try meditation for a half-hour each day as this has proven to be highly effective at reducing stress.

Another essential anti-stress strategy is to learn to recognize negative and self-defeating thoughts when they creep into your mind. Refuse to buy into them. Remind yourself that these kinds of thoughts are often triggered by fatigue, dehydration and improper eating habits.

Experts also recommend that you practice love, appreciation and gratitude at all times. Make a list of at least five things you are grateful for each day and keep these blessings in mind as you go through your daily routine.

All of these stress reduction techniques will help calm you down and keep you centered on all of the joy, beauty and future opportunities you have in your life. And, this in turn will minimize the over-production of stress hormones like cortisol that may be causing or contributing to your flare-ups. So find ways to stay stress-free to savor the smooth, clear skin you covet.

#23: Wear loose fitting clothing.

If you are prone to acne mechanica – which handymen, gardeners, musicians, athletes and other active people are - wear loose fitting clothes and 100% cotton fabrics. Do not wear belts, straps and helmets for a prolonged period.

Avoid synthetic fabrics such as nylon, as these fibers can aggravate acne by trapping moisture next to your skin. If you work out and sweat regularly, consider wearing some of the newer performance fabrics which help wick away moisture from the skin.

#24: Visualize being acne-free.

Another popular acne-fighting technique is called creative visualization. The first step is to relax and take a few deep breaths.

Envision how you would feel if you didn't have acne. Imagine your acne going away a little bit every day.

Your brain has a very powerful effect on your body. If your brain believes something, your body will come to believe it too.

Translation: if you think your acne will never go away – you're right. If you think your acne will go away – you're right too.

Every time you have a thought, you emit energy into your body and into the universe. If you continue to focus on your thoughts, your thoughts turn into actions. And your actions make your thoughts a reality. Doctors and other medical experts continue to be amazed at the mind-body connection: the fact that by believing you can heal, you can heal.

<u>How does this actually work?</u>

The hypothalamus, the emotional center of the brain, actually transforms your emotions into your body's unconscious physical responses. It does this by reading your emotions via your neuropeptides, the chemical messenger hormones, which carry your feelings back and forth between your body and your brain.

As the receptor and interpreter of your neuropeptides, the hypothalamus also controls your body's appetite, blood sugar levels, temperature, adrenal and pituitary glands, heart, lung, digestive and circulatory systems. And, it links your thought perceptions to each and every one of your bodily functions so that your body and your brain work together as one.

As a result, whether you have positive or negative thoughts, your brain totally accepts these thoughts without judgment... and sends these thoughts along to your body, which also accepts these thoughts without question. While positive thoughts and emotions have been shown to actually boost the immune system, negative thoughts and emotions have been shown to actually lower the immune system. So if you want positive results, think positive thoughts.

<u>How to put this powerful visualization tool to work for you.</u>

- Find a quiet place to sit or lie down.
- Get relaxed to access your subconscious mind.
- Center yourself by focusing on deep breathing.
- Totally relax your body and your mind.

- Visualize what you want.
- Think of or speak your intentions out loud.
- See yourself healing and as you want to be.
- Feel the healing taking place.
- Know the healing is being accomplished.
- "See" yourself becoming "acne-free" every single day.

By staying with your vision to become acne-free, you begin to make behavioral, dietary and other lifestyle choices that help manifest your goal over time.

Vitamin and Mineral Supplements

#25: Take a multi-vitamin.

Because most of us do not get all of the nutrients we need from the foods we eat, it is advisable to take a daily vitamin and mineral supplement. Acne, like many other medical conditions, can also be related to vitamin deficiencies. In addition, certain vitamin and mineral supplements have been shown to help alleviate acne, such as vitamins A, B, C, D, and magnesium, selenium and zinc.

You may be able to find a multi-vitamin or supplement that includes most or all of the essential acne-fighting vitamins and minerals listed below. If not, consider adding them as supplements to your multi-vitamin intake.

#26: Vitamin A.

Vitamin A is an essential vitamin traditionally used to help promote healthy skin and prevent acne outbreaks. It is also known for stimulating cell growth and healing the skin. Foods rich in vitamin A include chicken, turkey, butternut squash, lettuce, beetroot, peppers, milk and pork. Recommended daily allowance (RDA): 700 – 3,000 mcg.

#27: Thiamine (Vitamin B1)

Thiamine is an antioxidant that helps reduce the impact of free radicals on the skin, as well as facilitate the elimination of toxins from the body. Large amounts can be found in pork and organ meats. Other good dietary sources of thiamine include whole-grain or enriched cereals and rice, legumes, wheat germ, bran, brewer's yeast, and blackstrap molasses. Recommended daily allowance (RDA): 1.1 – 100 mg.

#28: Riboflavin (Vitamin B2)

Riboflavin plays an important role in the maintenance of healthy skin, hair and nails. In fact, acne is one of the symptoms of a riboflavin deficiency. In addition, when used in conjunction with vitamin A, riboflavin has been shown to help maintain and improve the mucous membranes in the digestive tract for a stronger immune system. Trace amounts of riboflavin can be found in beef, lamb liver, wild rice, pasta, soy milk, wholegrain cereals, yeast, pulses, seeds and dairy products.

Recommended daily allowance (RDA): 1.6 mg – 200 mg.

#29: Niacin (Vitamin B3).

Niacin improves blood circulation, which is necessary to stimulate healthy cell growth and enable the skin to repair itself after being ravaged by acne. Niacin is a primary vitamin that plays a critical role in the body's ability to metabolize protein, fat, and carbohydrates.
Niacin is also necessary to create red blood cells and hormones in the body, as well as to metabolize drugs and toxins.

When you factor in the many causes of acne, such as diet, hormones and stress, niacin packs a powerful punch in its ability to address all of these triggers at the same time. Foods rich in niacin include meat, fish, brewers yeast, nuts, seeds, soy beans, potatoes, dried fruit, tomatoes and peas. Milk, green leafy vegetables, coffee and tea also provide some niacin. Recommended daily allowance (RDA): 14 – 150 mg.

#30: Pantothenic Acid (Vitamin B5).

Pantothenic acid helps reduce stress, indirectly reducing acne, which stress is known to cause or aggravate. Also, according to a study published in 1995 by Dr. Lit-Hung Leung, vitamin B5 resolved acne and decreased pore size.
Dr. Leung found that without sufficient quantities of pantothenic acid, the body's essential carbohydrate and fat metabolizing enzyme, Acetyl coenzyme A or acetyl-CoA, will preferentially produce androgens.

Since CoA regulates both hormones and fatty acids, a deficiency in pantothenic acid allows fatty acids to build up and be excreted through the sebaceous glands, causing acne. Pantothenic acid can be found in peanuts, liver, kidney beans, avocado, mushrooms, seeds and other nuts, pumpkin, mushrooms, avocado, sweet potatoes, egg yolks, broccoli, dairy products, fish, chicken, wholegrain cereals, bread and bananas. Recommended daily allowance (RDA): 5 mg – 1,200 mg.

#31: Vitamin B6.

Vitamin B6 is involved in more bodily functions than almost any other single nutrient, and is particularly helpful in cases of acne, according to a study by Pennsylvania-based Dr. B. Leonard Snider. He noted that symptoms of acne were reduced by 50 – 75 percent with the use of vitamin B6. Vitamin B6 can be found in breakfast cereals (muesli, bran flakes and porridge oats), brown rice, brown bread, wheat germ, yeast, nuts, seeds, lentils, potatoes, baked beans, soy beans, bananas, white fish and meat. Recommended daily allowance (RDA): 1.3 – 100 mg.

#32: Vitamin C.

Vitamin C fights the effects of free radicals – environmental toxins that can wear down the body's immune system and have a damaging effect on the skin. It also works to remove the irritations and inflammations caused by acne, and engenders the regrowth of skin cells.

Vitamin C is present in fresh fruit, vegetables, fruit juices, kiwi, Brussels sprouts, and peppers. Recommended daily allowance (RDA): 75 – 2,000 mg.

#33: Vitamin E.

Vitamin E also helps counteract acne. It protects cells against the potentially harmful effects of free radicals, and also enhances healing and tissue repair.

Vitamin E can be found in vegetable oils, nuts, seeds, soy beans, beans, avocados, margarine, egg yolk, flour, whole grains and green leafy vegetables. Recommended daily allowance (RDA): 15 – 1,000 mg.

Vitamin E capsules can also be broken open and the liquid applied as a topical remedy to reduce the inflammation and redness of acne outbreaks and to speed the healing of acne-related scars.

#34: Calcium.

Calcium helps maintain the acid alkali balance of the blood, which is important for clear skin. It also helps the body absorb nutrients more effectively; and, it soothes the stomach, which can be irritated by essential nutrients such as zinc. Milk, yogurt, and cheese are rich natural sources of calcium. Non-dairy sources include vegetables, such as Chinese cabbage, kale, and broccoli. Recommended daily allowance (RDA): 1,000 - 1,300 mg.

#35: Magnesium.

Magnesium is known to help reduce inflammation, which is an approach often used to combat acne according to the American Academy of Dermatology. Excellent sources of magnesium include Swiss chard, spinach, summer squash, broccoli, blackstrap molasses, halibut, turnip greens, cucumber, green beans, celery, kale, and a variety of seeds including pumpkin, sunflower, sesame and flax. Recommended daily allowance (RDA): 300 – 900 mg.

#36: Selenium.

Selenium is beneficial for reducing inflammation and for alleviating chronic skin conditions such as eczema, acne and psoriasis. Its anti-inflammatory effects also benefit acne sufferers by reducing the appearance and severity of inflamed lesions. The best source of selenium is Brazil nuts. Other sources, which must be grown or raised under ideal soil conditions, are button and shiitake mushrooms, mustard seeds, barley and oats. Also, foods such as cod, halibut, salmon, shrimp, snapper, tuna, calf's liver, lamb, and turkey contain selenium. Recommended daily allowance (RDA): 55 – 400 mg.

#37: Zinc.

Zinc is an extremely powerful antioxidant that is essential to supporting the immune system as well as maintaining healthy skin, according to a recent study conducted at Duke University. Among the findings: "Zinc protects against UV radiation, enhances wound healing, contributes to immune and neuropsychiatric functions, and decreases the relative risk of cancer and cardio-vascular disease."

Good sources of zinc include: sea vegetables, spinach, pumpkin seeds, sesame seeds, summer squash, asparagus, collard and mustard greens, broccoli, peas, yogurt, shrimp, miso, and maple syrup. It is important to remember that zinc can create abdominal distress in some people if taken in doses above 100 mg per day. It can also cause nausea in some on an empty stomach. Recommended daily allowance (RDA): 15 – 80 mg.

#38: Fish Oil.

Studies have shown that increasing the amount of fish oil in your diet can help you treat your acne. The Omega-3 fatty acids in fish oil, particularly Eicosapenaenoic Acid, are believed to reduce inflammation, a major contributor to acne, by increasing the levels of anti-inflammatory Prostaglandins.

Omega-3's also help to stop the body from overproducing sebum, which is the main cause of acne breakouts. There is also a link between stress and the increased production of sebum. The good news is that the DHA in fish oil is a very effective mood regulator and stress minimizer – providing another sound reason to take fish oil for acne related problems.

Sources of fish oil naturally include most fish and seafood. In order to get the recommended dosage needed by the body, nutritionists recommend taking Omega-3 supplements, which are high in Eicosapenaenoic Acid, otherwise known as EPA. Recommended daily allowance (RDA): 1,000 – 3,000 mg.

Essential Herbs, Amino Acids and Antioxidants

Notes: The use of herbs is another time-honored way to strengthen the body's immune system and treat disease. Herbs, however, can interact with other herbs, supplements, or medications and trigger possible side effects in some individuals.

Also, if you are pregnant or nursing, the effects of different herbs upon your body and your baby are not fully known. For these reasons, you should take herbs with care and under the supervision of a health care provider if necessary.

#39: Burdock Root.

Burdock root is an herb that has been used for centuries to relieve a wide variety of epidermal aliments. According to Health911.com, "The herb burdock is effective in treating acne and is the most important herb for treating all forms of chronic skin problems."

Also, a 1967 German study published in the *Encyclopedia of Herbal Medicine* found that burdock root contains polyacetylenes, which have antifungal and antibiotic qualities to help fight acne-causing bacteria and other fungi that infect cracked skin. In addition, burdock root's diuretic action aids in eliminating impurities through the digestive system, rather than the skin where toxins can cause infections.

Not only does burdock root help improve the appearance of the skin, it also boosts immunity as well.

How to take burdock root. Capsules: 1 - 2 g, three times per day. Dried root: steep 2 - 6 grams in 150 ml (2/3 of a cup) in boiling water for 10 - 15 minutes and then strain and drink three times a day. As a tincture: (1:5): 2 - 8 mL 3 times per day; the tincture may also be applied to a cloth and wrapped around the affected skin area or wound. As a fluid extract: (1:1): 2 - 8 ml three times a day. And, as a tea: 2 - 6 grams steeped in 500 ml water (about 2 cups), three times per day.

Precautions: Pregnant or nursing women should avoid burdock as it may cause damage to the fetus. If you are sensitive to daises, chrysanthemums, or ragweed, you may also experience an allergic reaction to burdock. People who are dehydrated should not take burdock because the herb's diuretic effects may make dehydration worse.

It is best to avoid taking large amounts of burdock as a supplement because there are so few studies on the herb's safety. However, burdock eaten as a food is considered safe.

Because the roots of burdock closely resemble those of

belladonna or deadly nightshade (*Atropa belladonna*), there is a risk that burdock preparations may be contaminated with these potentially dangerous herbs. Be sure to buy products from established companies with good reputations. Do not gather burdock in the wild.

#40: Yellow Dock Root.

Yellow dock root has been used traditionally to aid digestion and to cleanse the blood and liver of toxins. Another one of its primary uses by herbalists is for skin conditions associated with poor digestion, poor liver function or "toxicity." The herb is known to treat acne, psoriasis and other skin blemishes, as well as to improve iron deficiency, reduce headaches, general irritability, and mental lethargy. Other wide-ranging applications include the treatment of anemia, anorexia, cramps, hepatitis, mouth sores and premenstrual syndrome (PMS).

How to take yellow dock root. There is no proven safe or effective dose for yellow dock in adults. Herbalists have recommended taking the roots and seeds daily for up to 12 months.

As a tincture of the fresh roots, 10-60 drops has been used (20 drops, two or three times a day). A fresh root vinegar preparation (1-2 tablespoons or 30 milligrams) has also been used. Based on expert opinion, no more than one cup (250 milligrams) of the dried seed tea should be taken per day.

Precautions: Like burdock root and many other herbs, yellow dock is not recommended for pregnant or nursing women. It may also cause mild diarrhea in some people. Yellow dock should also not be used if you have a history of kidney stones, liver disease, or an electrolyte abnormality, since the oxalates and tannins content in it may aggravate this condition.

#41: Horsetail Extract.

Horsetail extract has been used for both internal and external purposes since ancient times, according to the University of Maryland Medical Center. The main medicinal property of horsetail is its high silica content. This gives your cells strength, durability and flexibility and promotes collagen development in the skin. Horsetail also has antibacterial, antiseptic, and astringent properties. Due to these characteristics, horsetail is an effective treatment for damaged or problematic skin, including moderate to severe acne. It also has diuretic properties, and can help purge excess fluid and impurities from the body.

How to take horsetail extract: Horsetail extract that has standardized silica is recommended at 20 to 30 mg of silica daily, or 8 to 11 mg of silica per capsule. For external use, 10 teaspoons of powdered horsetail extract should be infused in about one quart of water.

Precautions: Do not take while pregnant, nursing or while you are on other diuretics or laxatives, or while drinking alcohol or with excessive amounts of licorice. Possible effects of taking excessive amounts of horsetail extract include an electrolyte imbalance and thiamine deficiency. Nicotine toxicity is possible, including symptoms of nausea, muscle weakness, fever and abnormal pulse rate.

#42: Green Tea Leaf Extract.

Green tea leaf extract is considered one of the most powerful antioxidants in the world. It has also been shown to possess antibiotic properties due to its ability to disrupt a specific stage of the bacterial DNA replication process. Also, according to a study by researchers at the University College London, green tea has the ability to lower hormone levels and correct imbalances, which have been shown to be a factor in the development of acne.

How to take green tea leaf extract: A dosage of 2 - 3 cups of green tea per day (for a total of 240 - 320 mg polyphenols) or 100 - 750 mg per day of standardized green tea extract is recommended.

Precautions: People with heart problems, kidney disorders, stomach ulcers, and psychological disorders (particularly anxiety) should not take green tea. Pregnant and breastfeeding women should also avoid green tea. Also, people who drink excessive amounts of caffeine (including caffeine from green tea) for prolonged periods of time may experience irritability, insomnia, heart palpitations, and dizziness.

#43: Grape Seed Extract.

Grape seed extract has been found to help regenerate damaged blood vessels and destroy bacteria in wounds, thus aiding in the healing process of acne and other skin conditions. These findings are based on a study funded by the National Institutes of Health and published in the Oct 12, 2002 issue of Free Radical Biology and Medicine.

How to take grape seed extract: Take 25 - 150 mg of a standardized extract (40 - 80% proanthocyanidins or 95% OPC value), 1 - 3 times daily.

Precautions: If you're pregnant or breast-feeding, you should not take grape seed extract without consulting with your physician or health care provider.

#44: Rose Hips Extract.

Rose hips extract is an abundant natural source of vitamin C, and also contains many other minerals and vitamins such as beta carotene, bioflavonoids, calcium, citrates, citric acid, iron malates, malic acid, niacin, phosphorus and vitamins A, B1, B2, E, K, and D. Studies have shown that the active ingredients found in rose hips can reduce inflammation and well as provide essential immune system support which aids in the defense and treatment of acne.

How to take rose hips extract: At this time, there is no precise scientific data regarding the appropriate dosage. Depending on your age and medical condition, since rose hips extract is essentially vitamin C, the recommended daily allowance (RDA) is: 75 – 2,000 mg.

Precautions: Rose hips are considered safe to take, but may cause allergic reactions in some people. However, if you are pregnant or breastfeeding, it is advisable not to take this extract without consulting with your doctor.

#45: Hydrolyzed Collagen.

Collagen is a highly digestible protein that helps firm and moisturize the skin. Two studies shown at a conference in Geneva, Switzerland showed that providing a daily supplement of hydrolyzed collagen improved both skin texture and appearance in 47 European women. The women who were given the hydrolyzed collagen treatment for aging, acne and dry skin experienced a 28 percent improvement in skin hydration levels as well as a 30 percent improvement in the reduction of fine lines and wrinkling.

<u>How to take hydrolyzed collagen:</u> A typical dose is 10 grams daily.

<u>Precautions:</u> Pregnant women and nursing mothers should avoid the use of hydrolyzed collagen. Those with renal or liver failure should also avoid this supplement. Experts also advise that you should check the source of the collagen to make sure that it is classified as carrying no detectable infectivity.

#46: L-Proline.

This is an amino acid that is important in the production of collagen and has been found to provide important benefits in acne and wound healing, cartilage building, and in flexible joint and muscle support. It has also been shown to help reduce the sagging, wrinkling, and aging of skin resulting from exposure to the sun and other skin conditions such as acne. Researchers believe L-Proline helps create healthy cells by breaking down protein, which is essential to both skin health and the creation of healthy connective and muscular tissue.

How to take L-Proline: You can take at least one gram per day in divided doses.

Precautions: If you are pregnant or nursing, you should consult with your doctor before taking, or avoid it all together on the side of caution.

#47: L-Lysine.

L-Lysine is one of eight essential amino acids and is instrumental in the formation of collagen, which supports the skin, muscles, and joints. It is also known to help repair and restore the elasticity of the skin during and after acne breakouts and other skin conditions.

How to take L-Lysine: The recommended dosage is 500 mg per day.

Precautions: If you are pregnant or nursing, you should consult with your doctor before taking, or avoid on the side of caution.

#48: Witch Hazel Extract

The American Indians are known to have used witch hazel medicinally due to its natural astringent properties.

Today, it is considered a useful supplement in fighting acne and promoting general skin health. In addition, many have found it to be the most helpful over-the-counter supplement in curbing facial sweating, which can also lead to acne. Witch hazel extract also has anti-inflammatory properties to help reduce redness in the skin caused by acne.

How to take witch hazel: Recommended oral dosage is two to three grams per day.

Precautions: If you are pregnant or nursing, you should consult with your doctor before taking, or avoid on the side of caution.

Other Natural Remedies and Topical Treatments

Acne has been around for centuries. So it's no surprise that the list of topical and other natural remedies is long and varied. From ingesting blackstrap molasses to dabbing apple cider vinegar, garlic oil, lemon juice, oatmeal, toothpaste and baking soda on to your blemishes to making a mask with avocadoes, honey and mayonnaise – there is no shortage of self-help solutions that have been tried over the years.

Here's a list of some of the most frequently mentioned remedies for your review. If you're not sure about your allergies, or if you're uncertain about the effect of one of these topical remedies on your face, try it on another area of your skin first to see the results.

#49: Salicylic acid and benzoyl peroxide.

Salicylic acid and benzoyl peroxide are both used for a topical treatment of acne and pimples. These chemical agents help fight against dermatological problems in different ways, with each exhibiting its own distinct properties.

Salicylic acid is an extract from the willow tree. As a beta-hydroxy acid, it is a colorless, crystalline, organic compound with an acidic base known to enhance the shedding of dead skin cells by acting as an exfoliating agent. Due to its exfoliating properties, it can help break-down whiteheads and blackheads, thereby helping the skin become clear. The acid penetrates the pores, reduces the pore size and wears away dead skin cells and enhances new cell growth.

The most common side effect of salicylic acid is dryness of the skin. It may cause a burning sensation, along with irritation.

Benzoyl peroxide, on the other hand, is organic peroxide. In contrast to salicylic acid, benzoyl peroxide inhibits and treats acne by killing the bacteria present in the skin and purifies the skin with its antiseptic properties. Similar to salicylic acid, it also removes dead cells, by acting as a peeling agent.

Like all peroxides, benzoyl peroxide is a potent bleaching agent and is also used in hair dyes. That's why it's a good idea to take precautions when applying benzoyl peroxide, as it has the potential to bleach almost instantly. Similar to salicylic acid, benzoyl peroxide causes dryness of the skin and induces a burning sensation on the skin. If using benzoyl peroxide dries your skin, then stop using it, as dry skin can exacerbate acne problems.

Salicylic acid is probably the choice for sensitive and dry skin, while benzoyl peroxide can provide an option for oily skin, as it reduces the skin bacteria and dries blemishes quickly. Benzoyl peroxide also has antiseptic properties, whereas salicylic acid is known for its mild to moderate effect in the treatment of acne.

#50: Apple Cider Vinegar.

Another highly regarded natural home remedy is the application of apple cider vinegar on the skin. Apply it evenly on your face after you have washed it thoroughly. The recommended application is to use a solution of two tablespoons of apple cider vinegar to one eight ounce glass of water, applied with a cotton ball several times a day, although less water can be used for a stronger solution. This will help reduce infection and dry out inflammation. Leave it on for twenty minutes and then wash off. As apple cider vinegar also has healing pro-perties and will act as both an astringent and a toner, if this remedy is followed regularly, it will contribute to making your skin clear of acne.

Another natural healing home remedy calls for the daily application of apple cider vinegar that has been infused with horseradish. Prepare a solution by adding two cups of ACV to one pound of grated horseradish. Let it sit for two weeks, then strain. Apple cider vinegar can also be taken internally to help resolve a wide variety of ailments.

#51: Witch Hazel.

Not only can witch hazel be taken internally, it is another time-tested topical solution for helping your skin fight acne bacteria and reduce redness. It is advisable to be careful with witch hazel as it can dry or irritate sensitive skin.

Witch hazel has antibacterial properties due to its tannin acid. As a result, it can help reduce the inflammation caused by acne and pimple production. Furthermore, tannin acid is a strong astringent, as the American Indians originally discovered, making it ideal for skin cleansing. Witch hazel is known to cause little to no allergic reactions.

Another plus is that witch hazel does not disrupt the pH balance of your skin. Also, it is very inexpensive and very easy to use. Simply soak a cotton ball with witch hazel solution and apply it on the affected areas of your skin; much like using a regular astringent. You can do this twice a day, but any more than that may cause irritation.

#52: Aloe Vera.

The watery gel from the aloe vera plant is another highly effective natural treatment for acne. The enzyme-rich gel has very soothing anti-inflammatory and antibacterial properties. It can also be taken internally and helps clean up and detox the digestive tract. This in turn can help clear up the skin.

Consistent and regular use of aloe vera can significantly improve symptoms of acne and the scarring from it. Aloe vera contains polysaccharides that serve as the building blocks for skin repair. Aloe vera can also help heal the wounds caused by acne by decreasing inflammation and reducing scarring.

Try applying 100% aloe vera gel to your acne-ravaged areas, either as a spot treatment or an overall moist-urizer. You can also use aloe vera gel as a facial mask. Spread it evenly and generously on your face before going to bed and let it stay overnight. Wash it off with warm water the morning after.

#53: Tea Tree Oil.

Tea tree oil is yet another popular and proven effective way to fight acne, and like apple cider vinegar, gives you a potent natural alternative to salicylic acid and benzoyl peroxide.

Tea tree oil originates from the Melaleuca alternifoliais tree in Australia. The reason it is very effective against acne is that it contains antifungal and antibacterial fighting substances called terpenes. Acne is often caused by bacteria and the terpenes either kill bacteria outright or weaken them enough to be destroyed by protective antibodies. Remember that pure tea tree oil is very strong and may cause you to suffer an allergic reaction if you place this oil directly on to your skin. You will need to dilute it depending on your skin type. For example, if you have oily skin, take a tablespoon of tea tree oil and mix it with nine tablespoons of water.

If your skin is a little sensitive, try mixing the tea tree oil with aloe vera gel instead of water. The gel will help neutralize any possible reactions you may have to the tea tree oil.

Before you use the tea tree solution, wash your face with a mild cleanser first. With a cotton ball, apply the solution to form a thin layer on your skin. When it's dry, you may want to put on a moisturizer (preferably oil-free).

#54: Olive Oil.

Put oil on oily skin? Yes. Not only is extra virgin olive oil an ideal source of healthy fats in your diet, it can also be used quite effectively as a natural moisturizer and mask to help create beautiful skin and alleviate breakouts.

First, rinse your face with warm water, then massage a small quantity of virgin olive oil into your skin until all the oil is absorbed. Then dab your face with a clean cloth until it mats the oily look. You can also add a few drops of olive oil to your moisturizer or face mask to give it an extra moisturizing and acne-fighting punch.

#55: Coconut Oil.

The health benefits of coconut oil are well documented,

and include hair care, skin care, stress relief, weight loss, increased immunity, proper digestion and metabolism. These benefits can be attributed to the presence of lauric acid, capric acid and caprylic acid, and their antimicrobial, antioxidant, antifungal, and antibacterial properties.

Coconut oil is excellent moisturizer for all types of skin without any adverse side effects. It is also very effective in treating a variety of skin infections and problems including psoriasis, dermatitis, eczema, acne and other conditions. It also delays wrinkles and sagging skin, which normally becomes more pronounced with age.

No wonder coconut oil, like aloe vera, forms the basic ingredient of various products such as soaps, lotions, and creams used for skin care. Use coconut oil as a moisturizer and mask like olive oil with noticeable results. Another benefit: coconut oil also helps relieve stress and makes your hair healthier and shiny. You can even cook with coconut oil to experience many of its health-promoting properties internally.

#56: Lavender Oil.

Apply a drop of this oil onto your affected areas and watch the healing begin. Many claim that lavender oil will help you get rid of your acne fast. Lavender also has well-known aromatherapy properties and its pleasing smell is said to help reduce stress.

As with all essential oils, lavender oil should be diluted with another oil such as jojoba or olive oil or with witch hazel before applying it to the skin.

#57: Jojoba Oil.

Similar to lavender oil, jojoba oil is another popular acne treatment that has stress-reducing effects as well. Jojoba oil is non-comedogenic, so it also makes an excellent skin-friendly moisturizer and can also be mixed with rosehips oil in a 5:2 proportion and applied to blemishes for a fast-acting anti-acne mask.

#58: Patchouli Oil.

Patchouli oil is from the puchaput perennial plant native to India and Malaysia. It is known to be very effective in softening rough, cracked and overly dehydrated skin and is widely used to treat acne, eczema, sores, ulcers, any fungal infections, as well as scalp disorders.

On the skin, this rich musky-sweet smelling oil is one of the most active tissue regenerators known as it helps to stimulate the growth of new skin cells. In wound healing, it cools down inflammation, resolves fungal and bacterial infections and promotes faster healing. Patchouli oil also helps prevent scarring when wounds or outbreaks heal.

Patchouli oil also has a grounding and balancing effect on your emotions, and is said to banish fatigue while sharpening the wits, fighting depression and alleviating anxiety.

#59: Camphor Oil with Caster Oil and Almond Oil.

Camphor oil comes from the Camphor tree native to China and Japan. It is an integral ingredient in many

Ayurvedic medicines for strengthening the heart, relieving knee and joint pain and revitalizing and rejuvenating the skin.

Rich in antioxidants, camphor oil is also very popular in treating acne and maintaining the overall health of the skin.

Camphor oil can be combined with almond and castor oil for a very simple and effective home remedy for acne. Mix half a cup of castor oil with half a cup of almond oil. Add one teaspoon of camphor oil. Shake the mixture well. Before you apply it to your skin, wash your face and pat dry. Leave this oil on your skin overnight for better results.

Another treatment idea is to wash your face gently to remove the impurities, then apply a hot compress or use steam for about 20 minutes to open the pores on your face. Then gently massage the camphor oil onto your skin.

#60: Blackstrap Molasses.

Blackstrap molasses is known for its many healing properties and many report a reduction of acne breakouts after taking two to four tablespoons each day. It can also be used as a moisturizer to help soothe and replenish dry acne-ravaged skin.

#61: Baking Soda.

Pour a small amount of baking soda on your palm. Mix it

with a few drops of water. Apply it on your face. Let it stay there for about 15 - 20 minutes, and then rinse with water. Use this face mask for acne twice a week. According to a countless number of acne sufferers, your skin will feel softer and look clearer before you know it.

#62: Lemon Juice.

Lemon juice is probably one of the most under-rated herbal remedies, although its use as topical treatment for acne is highly regarded.

Used for centuries for its healing and therapeutic properties, lemon juice exhibits a strong antibacterial effect on the body. In fact, experiments have shown that the bacteria indigenous to malaria, cholera, diphtheria, typhoid and other deadly diseases are destroyed in lemon juice.

Lemon juice is also known for its high natural vitamin C level, which has been shown to be far more powerful than the synthetic variety. This exceptional potency is due in part to the synergistic effect created by the combination of vitamin C with the wealth of bioflavonoids in lemon juice. Lemon juice also contains niacin, thiamin and vitamin A – vitamins that are recognized for their ability to fight acne.

Include lemon juice in your recipes and diet, and be sure to dab a drop or two on to your breakouts to reduce redness and swelling. As pure lemon juice can be a bit too strong for some skin, try diluting it with a little water first.

#63: Garlic.

Garlic can be used both internally and externally in your quest for clear, radiant skin. Garlic is considered by many to be an herbal "wonder drug", with a storied reputation for preventing everything from acne to the common cold.

High in sulfur compounds, selenium, manganese, and vitamin B, garlic has been shown to reduce inflammation, and has antibacterial and antiviral properties. Garlic is also a very powerful natural antibiotic, and works across a broad-spectrum of medical conditions. Better still, the bacteria in the body do not appear to develop a resistance to garlic's antibiotic powers as they do with today's pharmaceutical antibiotics. This means that its positive health benefits can continue over time rather than helping to breed antibiotic resistance.

Research has also established that garlic, especially aged garlic, can have a very potent antioxidant effect on the body. Among other things, it protects cells against damaging free radicals that contribute to acne, as well as numerous other physical ailments.

Furthermore, studies have shown that consuming just two cloves of fresh garlic per day can help your body ward off and defend against certain types of infections, especially those of the skin that can lead to acne.

In terms of dosage strength, a stronger tasting clove has more sulfur content, and therefore more potential medicinal value. Some people have suggested that organically grown garlic tends toward an even higher sulfur level and, as a result, provides even greater health benefits.

While garlic can be eaten or taken in capsule form, it also provides a highly-recommended topical treatment for even the most severe breakouts, due in part to its sulfur content. Crush some garlic and squeeze the juice from the bulb on to your affected areas. It may smell a bit strong, but many swear by this odiferous antibacterial, antibiotic and anti-inflammatory acne-fighting treatment.

A final note of caution, some people are allergic to garlic and can experience skin rashes, fever and headaches when exposed to the bulb. Make sure you're not one of them before you try this treatment.

#64: Basil.

Take 10 to 12 tablespoons of basil and put it into boiling water for about two hours. After the liquid cools off, apply it to your face for 20 - 30 minutes. Then lay a cool damp towel over this area for about 10 minutes.

#65: Wet Tea Bag.

Wipe or hold a cool used tea bag over your acne areas to help reduce pain, redness and swelling.

The tannic acid in the wet tea leaves helps soothe the skin's soreness and inflammation. A wet tea bag is also known to help soothe the sting of a sunburn and other burns to the skin.

#66: Honey.

Another effective way to fight acne is to put raw or natural honey on your face several times per day. Honey has antiseptic, antioxidant and antibacterial properties to inhibit acne bacterial growth, reduce acne-related inflammation and promote healing.

Let the honey dry for 20 minutes or so, then rinse with warm water. Some have found that it will make pimples go away within weeks. Honey will also give your skin a smoother, silkier, healthier glow. And, it is known to be very effective at fading and removing scars.

#67: Honey and Avocado Mask.

Mix a mask of equal parts of honey and a mashed-up avocado and apply it on to your acne areas. Leave it on for 20 – 25 minutes, then rinse with warm water.

#68: Honey and Apple Mask.

Grate half of an apple and mix it up with about four teaspoons of honey. Put it on your blemishes and let it sit for at least 20 minutes, then rinse. As with other honey masks, this treatment is known to prevent and alleviate breakouts, heal dry skin and leave your skin with a more radiant look.

#69: Honey and Cinnamon Mask.

This is another one of the most recommended topical treatments for acne. Mix one or two teaspoons of cinnamon with three or four teaspoons of honey and apply it to your acne.

Leave this paste on as long as possible, including overnight if you can. Then, rinse with warm water.

When ingested, a mixture of honey and cinnamon is also considered to be a very effective method for strengthening the immune system and resolving a long list of health ailments including indigestion, bladder infections, bad breath and the common cold.

#70: Honey, Cinnamon, Lemon Juice and Nutmeg Mask.

Here's another natural mask to try. Mix two parts honey to one part cinnamon and lemon juice, with a dash of nutmeg. Apply to acne areas for 20 – 30 minutes, then rinse with warm water.

#71: Plain Natural Yogurt Mask.

After you've taken a hot shower and your pores are opened up, apply some plain natural yogurt on to your face, back and other acne areas.

Leave it on for 20 - 25 minutes, then rinse. Try this treatment daily for several weeks.

#72: Yogurt and Strawberry Mask.

Mix plain natural yogurt with mashed strawberries and apply as a mask. Leave on for at least 20 minutes, then rinse.

#73: Tomato Pulp, Honey and Rose Water Mask.

Before bathing, put a mixture of real, not packaged, tomato pulp or paste and honey with a few drops of rose water on to your face and keep it on for at least 20 minutes before washing off.

#74: Cream, Glycerin and Lemon Juice Mask.

Before going to bed at night, put a mixture of cream, glycerin, and lemon juice on your face and keep it on for a short while before washing.

#75: Toothpaste.

Toothpaste doesn't just help clean your teeth, it can help clean up your acne and lessen the redness associated with your outbreaks. Dab a spot of toothpaste on to your pimples and leave on until it dries. Then wash it off with cold water. Follow up with a soothing non-comedogenic moisturizer.

#76: Baking Soda, Banana, Honey, Sour Cream, and Maple Syrup Mask.

Another topical remedy involves mixing baking soda with one banana mashed up, 1/2 cup of sour cream, 1/4 cup of maple syrup, and 3/4 cup of honey. Mix these ingredients together and apply to your face and other acne areas. Leave on as long as you can after it dries, then rinse it off with warm water.

#77: Miracle Whip or Mayonnaise Mask.

This is yet another natural mask to try. Leave it on for 20 – 30 minutes, then rinse.

#78: Tomato Sauce, Lemon Juice and Toothpaste Mask.

Mix up a paste using these ingredients, with two parts tomato sauce to one part each lemon juice and toothpaste. Apply it to your breakouts and leave it on as long as possible – overnight if feasible.

#79: Baking Soda, Cinnamon, Honey, Lemon and Nutmeg Mask.

Another popular topical treatment involves mixing about three teaspoons each of baking soda and lemon juice with at least two tablespoons of honey. Add in a bit of nutmeg and at least a half a teaspoon of cinnamon. Mix it all together, put it on your acne, and leave it on for about an hour and a half. Then wash off with warm water.

#80: Oatmeal Mask.

Oatmeal is another popular topical treatment for acne due to its soothing and healing properties. Boil 1/2 cup of oatmeal in water. Let it cool, then spread a thick layer on to your breakouts. Leave it on for at least 15 - 20 minutes, then rinse.

#81: Oatmeal, Lemon Juice and Yogurt Mask.

Mix one tablespoon of cooked oatmeal and one table-spoon of plain natural yogurt together. Add a few drops of lemon juice. Apply this paste on to your face and leave it on for 10 - 25 minutes. Then rinse with cold water.

This mask has also been reported to work well for reducing acne scars. Try it at least three times per week to help control your acne.

#82: Sandalwood Powder.

Mix sandalwood powder with a few drops of rose water, or mix it in equal parts with olive, lavender, coconut or tea tree oil to form a mask. Leave the mask on until it dries for smoother, brighter skin.

#83: Almond, Milk, Orange Juice and Vitamin A Mask.

Soak 10 almonds overnight. Crush them up and add three tablespoons of milk, two tablespoons of orange juice and the contents of two vitamin A tablets. Apply this paste to your face for 20 - 30 minutes each day to get rid of acne and promote healthy skin.

#84: White and Brown Sugar.

Mix two parts white sugar with one part brown sugar. Add enough water to form a paste, and apply it to your acne areas. Leave it on for 20 - 30 minutes and then rinse. This will help rid your skin of acne and foster a more lustrous complexion.

#85: Egg Whites.

Another recommended acne remedy is to apply some egg whites on to your skin for 20 - 30 minutes, then rinse. Proponents of this treatment promise your skin will regain its clear radiant glow.

#86: Turmeric Powder and Mint.

Still another popular mask involves mixing these two spices together with water to form a paste and putting it on to your blemishes. Regular application is said to reduce acne outbreaks and promote smoother skin.

#87: Ice Massage.

Gently applying ice will reduce swelling and redness due to acne. Be careful not to push the ice into your skin as this may damage your skin cells.

#88: Tomato and Cucumber Juice.

Mix equal parts of these juices and put them on your blemished areas. Leave on for at least 20 minutes to tighten your pores and reduce redness.

#89: Lemon Juice and Rose Water.

Mix in equal parts and apply for at least 25 minutes, then rinse.

#90: Neem Leaves.

Margosa leaves, more popularly known as neem, provide another one of the most recommended and potent healers of skin problems like acne. Crush these leaves in a blender, then add in some turmeric powder and apply this on to your skin. Let it dry and then wash off.

Many report that this treatment will get rid of the excess oil as well as the accumulated dirt on your face. Another option is to introduce neem leaves into your bath water to help cleanse the whole body and prevent the onset of acne.

#91: Grapefruit Seed Extract.

Grapefruit seed extract acts as a cleanser and removes oil and dirt from your skin. You can also take 2 - 3 drops of grapefruit extract and mix it with one tablespoon of water and apply this solution on to your blemishes with cotton balls. Wash off after 10 - 15 minutes or so, and pat dry.

#92: Calamine Lotion.

Calamine lotion helps to dry up acne breakouts without damaging your skin. It works in a similar fashion as benzoyl peroxide, but is far less harsh. It gently clears up acne breakouts while improving the texture of the skin.

You can apply calamine lotion directly on to your face using a cotton swab. Leave it on overnight, if possible, and then rinse it off the next morning. Numerous acne sufferers report that you will see a noticeable change in your acne within a matter of days.

#93: Epsom Salt.

Epsom salt, otherwise known as magnesium sulphate, is a mineral that occurs naturally with a myriad of medicinal uses, especially for acne. Not only is it an anti-inflammatory, it can also be used to reduce skin irritation and redness.

To help get rid of acne outbreaks, dissolve about two tablespoons of Epsom salt in a cup of water. Dip a cotton ball or hand-towel into this solution and gently place it on your acne areas. Keep this on for 15 - 20 minutes, and then rinse.

You can also add about two cups of Epsom salt, along with a few drops of an essential oil, to your tub to create a relaxing bath. Soaking your body in this mixture will not only reduce acne and help detoxify your skin, it will also make your skin softer and smoother.

For an exfoliating scrub, add a tablespoon of Epsom salt to oatmeal and use this to gently wash your face. Be sure to apply a moisturizer after patting your face dry.

#94: Mix and Match and Make up Your Own Mask.

Many of the natural ingredients listed in this book have also been mixed up in an astonishing array of different combinations.

From combining mashed up apples, bananas, and almonds with tomato sauce, yogurt, oatmeal, and honey to adding varying amounts of olive, lavender, tea tree and jojoba oils to combining lemon, cucumber and carrot juices... there is hardly a combination of ingredients that hasn't been tried.

However, before trying any of your mixed and matched masks on your face, apply them to another less noticeable acne area on your body to make sure they work without over-drying or creating an allergic reaction on your skin.

#95: Finally, keep your acne in perspective.

Not only can acne damage your skin, it can devastate your self-esteem and destroy your self-confidence. Don't let it.

The appearance of acne can cause a great deal of trauma in many people, particularly teenagers and young adults.

This only elevates existing levels of anxiety and stress, which further irritates the skin and worsens acne related problems. What's worse, this self-perpetuating cycle remains persistent unless and until you can get your anxiety levels regarding your acne under control.

Stay positive and be patient in your journey to become acne free. For example, if you constantly find yourself thinking "my acne will never go away", ask yourself if this thought is really true. It's not. Your acne will go away, maybe not as soon or as quickly as you'd like.

But it will go away!

So don't let your breakouts interfere with believing in yourself. Don't let your blemishes prevent you from setting a good example, pursuing your interests with passion, or making a difference in the lives of your loved ones and your community.

You have the power to make your acne go away and stay away for good. So get started today – and start enjoying the clear, smooth, radiant skin you deserve.

If you think you can do it, you're absolutely right!

Frequently Asked Questions

1. What is acne?

Commonly known as blemishes, pimples or zits – acne is an outbreak of red, pus-filled eruptions caused primarily by bacterial attacks on the skin. Acne usually appears on the face and shoulders, and also may occur on other parts of the body.

And, if you thought acne was a teen problem, think again! It affects men and women in their twenties, thirties, forties and sometimes even as late as fifties! While there are several different forms of acne, and a wide variety of causes and aggravating factors, acne is almost always physically noticeable and psychologically unnerving – at any age.

2. What causes acne?

Although it seems like pimples and other forms of acne appear virtually overnight, breakouts involve a rather extended process at the cellular level.

Acne on the face or anywhere else on the body can be caused by a number of different reasons such as: excess sebum production by the skin, developmental and physiological changes occurring during the teenage years, a hormonal imbalance, genetics, allergies to certain foods, usage of the wrong kind of cosmetics, stress and other lifestyle and/or dietary factors.

Excess sebum production by the skin.

The main reason behind acne appearing on the skin is excess sebum production. The hair and skin on the body are kept lubricated with the help this oily liquid, which is secreted or produced by what is known as the sebaceous glands. Now this sebum liquid, after it is secreted, makes it way through the sebum, and reaches the skin through a pore or opening of the hair follicle.

From a medical perspective, acne erupts when pores, which are microscopic-sized holes in the skin, become clogged. Each pore is an opening to a follicle, which has an oil gland to help lubricate the skin and remove old skin cells. When these glands produce too much oil, the pores can become blocked.

Along with this, the body can also produce an excess of dead skin cells, which also causes pores to become backed up. This allows bacteria and inflammatory cells to build up, creating a blockage called a plug.

The top of the plug may be white (a whitehead) or dark (a blackhead). If this plug breaks open, the bacteria inside causes swelling and red bumps to form, known as papules and pustules. If the inflammation is deep in the skin, the pimples may enlarge to form hard cysts that are also painful.

Another factor to consider is that there are more seba-ceous glands on the facial area than any other part of the body. The chest and back are the other two areas where these oil glands can be found in a fairly large number, resulting in more acne breakouts on these areas as well.

Being a teenager.

During the teen years, there is often an increase in the production of the testosterone hormone, as well as an increase in the production of sebum by the sebaceous glands; and many believe this is one of the main reasons acne is so prevalent in teenagers.

Hormonal Changes and Imbalances.

Another cause of acne is the hormonal changes that take place in the body during puberty and during the female menstruation cycle. Acne can also flare up when a woman is pregnant or is entering menopause.

Hormone changes are one of the most common causes of acne breakouts. These mostly occur during puberty as the body goes through numerous hormonal changes, and as a result, this causes acne breakouts. Acne flare-ups during pregnancy are also common as the body goes through a rush of hormonal changes. Hormonal acne is not only found during pregnancy but also affects women of all ages and is most evident during their menstrual cycle

Certain hormones in the body, such as androgens and testosterone, stimulate the sebaceous glands, thus causing an increase in the amount of oil produced by these glands. When the skin becomes oily due to hormonal imbalance in the body, the skin pores get clogged, resulting in acne outbreaks.

Hormonal imbalance induced acne is commonly experienced by women during menstruation, pregnancy, perimenopause and menopause. While in men, it is most prominent during the teen years.

Heredity.

Acne can be hereditary too, and is known to run in families. Those with a history of acne problems in the family are more likely to have acne breakouts. If your parents had acne, chances are you will too. The good news, however, is that there haven't been any conclusive studies regarding this. So you might get away with an occasional pimple, even if acne is an issue with other members of your family.

Medicines.

Another acne trigger is the intake of certain medicines, which can increase the incidence of acne in some people. Birth control pills, steroids, hormonal therapies and many other medicines can trigger acne.

Overuse or Wrong Use of Cosmetics.

If you use certain cosmetics such as make-up, shampoo or face creams which are unsuitable for your skin type – this can also trigger an acne attack.

For example, if you already have acne-prone skin and you use oily or greasy creams or other cosmetic products, these can clog your pores and result in acne. Not just that, but the chemical compounds in certain cosmetic products can also aggravate or cause acne breakouts.

Stress.

Clinical studies suggest that stress can also cause of breakouts, and increase the severity of them as well. Stress induces the adrenal glands to produce more hormones and also slows down the healing process of acne, which means it stays for a prolonged period.

Stress increases the supply of adrenaline in the blood, a hormone present in both males and females. This leads to increased levels of the hormone 'cortisol' secreted in your body which disrupts its hormonal balance. Excessive adrenaline reduces the nutrient-absorbing capacity of the body and directly attacks our largest organ, the skin.

When your body is under stress, its immunity to fight foreign bodies decreases significantly. This reduces the ability of the body to heal by 40 percent. The time taken for acne to clear up naturally slows down dramatically, which increases the appearance of acne and leaves the skin with unsightly blemishes.

Also, during stress, the nervous system stimulates the production of excess sebum, containing the corticotropin-releasing hormone (CRH), which is the primary reason for hair loss, clogged pores, and oily skin. And this, of course, also aggravates acne problems.

Interestingly, at least 90% people under stress have re-ported acne related-problems.

<u>Food allergies.</u>

In the past several years, numerous studies have emerged concluding that the link between milk and acne is strong, with one study even finding a 44% higher incidence of severe acne among those who drink two or more glasses of milk a day. This particular study, conducted in 2005, found the strongest association for skim milk intake, suggesting that the hormones and other allergenic proteins found in milk can increase sebum production and inflammation.

Other foods that may cause or contribute to acne include red meat, eggs, grains, processed foods and caffeine.

<u>Unhealthy Diet and Lifestyle choices.</u>

Eating processed foods and consuming unhealthy drinks, such as soda which has no nutritional value, are two more factors that can aggravate acne breakouts around mouth or on the face.

Despite the commonly held belief that chocolate, nuts, and greasy foods cause acne, research does not confirm this notion. Diets high in refined sugars may be related to acne however.

Improper hygiene can also cause or aggravate acne. If the skin is not maintained and cleaned regularly, dirt enters into the pores and prevents the skin from receiving adequate oxygen for nourishment, resulting in skin conditions such as acne breakouts.

Irregular sleeping patterns or lack of sleep can also play a major role in aggravating acne as lack of sleep results in hormonal changes that could affect the skin.

Other factors that can aggravate acne are excess sweating, friction from hats, helmets or backpacks on the skin and insulin resistance.

Action Plan:
Okay. So what do you think is causing your acne?
Put a check next to your potential acne triggers.

__ Being a teenager
__ Hormonal changes and imbalances
__ Heredity
__ Medicines
__ Overuse or wrong cosmetics
__ Product sensitivity, such as to soaps, etc.
__ Stress
__ Food Allergies
__ Unhealthy diet and lifestyle

3. What are the types of acne?

There are several different kinds of acne - depending on the type of plug created by the build up of oil and dead skin cells that accumulate in the hair follicle. Here's a list of the most common forms of acne.

Type	Characteristics
Whitehead	The soft plug that forms as a result of the accumulation of excess sebum and dead skin cells: May be totally blocked, with a white appearance.
Blackhead	When the soft plug is partially, but not completely blocked, it remains open at the skin surface. This causes the melanin of the skin to react with oxygen, making the plug darken over time.
Pustules	This type of acne develops as bumps, which are typically red and tender to touch. These remain inflamed, and have a white or yellow center.
Papules	Like pustules, papules indicate infection or inflammation in the hair follicles. They also surface as small, red bumps, which can also be tender to the touch.
Nodules	In some cases, the excess sebum and dead skin cells start building up deep beneath the surface of the hair follicles. When this happens, it causes the formation of lumps, which are sometimes large and almost always painful.
Cysts	This type of acne is the most severe and painful. Like nodules, cysts form beneath the skin's surface in the form of lumps. These pimples get filled with pus however, and this is what increases the risk of acne scars.
Acne Conglobata	A combination of pustules and nodules, this form of acne is also severe and is known to affect areas such as the back, buttocks, chest, shoulders, upper arms, and thighs – as well as the face.

Another form of acne, called acne mechanica, develops due to the friction caused by headwear, clothing or sports equipment. The presence of a belt, strap, synthetic fiber, helmet or shoulder pads – along with the sweat that is caused beneath the material – makes the skin vulnerable to acne. This type of acne can develop at any age and may appear not only on the face, but shoulders, back, waist, legs, under the arms or in the groin area.

Action Plan:
What kind of acne do you have?

__ Whiteheads
__ Blackheads
__ Pustules
__ Papules
__ Nodules
__ Cysts
__ Acne Mechanica

All of these forms of acne will respond positively to the tips listed in this book.

4. How many people have acne?

Over 60 million Americans suffer from acne, including over 75 percent of teens, according to the American Dermatological Association. This makes acne is the most common skin condition in the United States. Acne can happen at any age, even in infants. In addition, people in their 30s, 40s and 50s may also have acne.

5. What is the impact of acne?

Although acne is not a life-threatening condition, it can be very painful. In addition, it can have a very damaging psychological impact on those who suffer from it.

If you're a teenager, acne can be especially problematic. That's because it appears at the moment in your life when you're super self-conscious about your looks and want to fit in. Teenagers with acne are often susceptible to depression and often show poor self-esteem and a general lack of confidence.

These issues are also common for young adults, although perhaps not to the same degree. The large incidence of acne is the reason there are so many skin products in the market, designed to fight, treat, and hopefully help make it disappear.

6. Is there a cure for acne?

Unfortunately, there is no known cure for acne at this time. There are literally dozens of natural treatments and remedies for acne however, some more effective than others.

In addition, there are a wide variety of prescription medications available, but many have known side effects.

After careful research, we've compiled a list of natural treatments and remedies that have little or no side effects, starting on page five.

7. Will my acne go away naturally?

In most cases, the answer is yes. Acne usually goes away after the teenage years, but it may last into middle age. The condition often responds well to treatment after six to eight weeks, but it may flare up from time to time. Maintaining a healthy lifestyle and diet can make a dramatic difference.

8. Should I take prescription drugs for acne?

Acne is a medical condition and caused by a variety of factors inside your body. So it is only natural that you would want to visit with your doctor, dermatologist or other health care professional regarding the source or cause of your breakouts – and what your treatment alternatives are.

It is also only natural that your doctor may prescribe a short course of antibiotics to attack the acne-related bacteria that is attacking your skin.

However, just because your doctor or dermatologist may prescribe these medications does not mean they are harmless. While these chemicals may offer short-term relief to your condition, some of the documented reactions to these drugs can be downright dangerous and even deadly.

The question is: what are you willing to risk to be acne-free? If you are considering or currently taking prescription medication, such as antibiotics or Accutane, you should be aware of the possible side effects that come from using these drugs.

From nausea, vomiting, diarrhea, sun sensitivity and yeast infections to liver and kidney damage, birth defects, depression and suicide – the consequences of taking prescription drugs for acne range from mildly discomforting to totally devastating.

That is why it is important to ask your health care provider for safer alternatives to prescription medications and the nutritional guidance needed to help you get rid of your acne naturally and without any unnecessary risks.

How antibiotics work. They kill the bad bacteria.

Antibiotics work in several ways. First, they decrease the bacteria in and around the acne follicle and reduce the irritating chemicals produced by white blood cells. They also reduce the concentration of free fatty acids in the sebum, also minimizing your body's inflammatory response. The most frequently used antibiotics for acne include:

<u>Oral antibiotics for acne include:</u>

Tetracycline
Erythromycin
Minocycline (also known as Minocin)
Doxycycline
Clindamycin
Lymecycline (also known as Tetralysal)

Tetracycline is the most widely prescribed antibiotic for acne. The main drawback for this antibiotic is that it must be taken on an empty stomach to be the most effective. For a teenager who eats frequently, this can be challenging. Tetracycline is also known to cause gastrointestinal distress and candida vaginal yeast infections in women, and it should not be given to pregnant women or children under 9 years of age.

Erythromycin is also a very commonly prescribed antibiotic for acne. It has several advantages over tetracycline. First, it has anti-inflammatory properties that help reduce redness in lesions, in addition to killing bacteria. Also, it can and should be taken with food - a benefit for teenagers. It can cause stomach upset and nausea, but can be used by pregnant women.

Minocycline is a tetracycline derivative and used for decades as a treatment for acne, especially for pustular acne. While the absorption of minocycline also decreases with food, it is not as dramatic as the decrease seen with tetracycline. Major side effects include dizziness, nausea, vomiting, skin pigmentation changes, and tooth dis-coloration. The skin and tooth changes are seen more often in those who have taken this drug for a long time.

Doxycycline is often prescribed to people who do not respond to or cannot tolerate erythromycin or tetracycline. Unlike the tetracycline drugs, doxycycline should be taken with food, otherwise it can cause severe nausea. Doxycycline is also more likely than the tetracycline drugs to increase sensitivity to the sun, or cause sunburns.

Clindamycin is used as an oral antibiotic for acne, but it is most widely prescribed as a topical antibiotic. The major side effect of clindamycin therapy is a serious intestinal infection called pseudomembranous colitis caused by the bacteria, Clostridium difficile.

Lymecycline or Tetralysal is not recommended for pregnant women, those who are breastfeeding and those who have lupus or liver disease. Some of the common side effects of Lymecycline are headache, nausea, vomiting and diarrhea.

Antibiotics also kill the "good" bacteria in your body, and possible side effects can be severe.

All prescription medications come with the risk of side effects.

Antibiotics kill off all of the bacteria in your body, in-cluding the good bacteria your body needs to complete the digestion process and maintain a strong immune system.

Wiping out the good bacteria also causes yeast to grow in

both men and women, including candida vaginal yeast infections in women. Tetracycline seems to cause these side effects most often.

In addition, all oral antibiotics can also lessen the effectiveness of birth control pills; and many adult acne sufferers have acne as a direct result of using or over-using antibiotics or contraceptive pills to treat their acne when they were teenagers.

23 possible side effects of using antibiotics for acne:
Nausea and vomiting
Diarrhea
Sun sensitivity
Yeast infections, which cause:
Fatigue
Bloating
Mood Swings
Anxiety
Depression
Thrush
Cystitis
IBS
Loss of appetite
Skin discoloration
Tooth discoloration (yellow teeth)
Dry "leather-like" skin
Sore mouth
Difficulty in swallowing
Inflamed colon
Inflamed pancreas
Rash
Headache
Ear noises and temporary deafness

Even with good nutrition, it can take time to get your body chemistry back to normal after taking antibiotics.

The most dangerous acne treatment of all:
Retinoids such as Accutane.

Accutane is a prescription medication used to treat severe, disfiguring acne that has not responded to other treatments such as topical creams and antibiotics.

Manufactured by Hoffman-LaRoche and approved by the FDA in 1982, Accutane, generically known as isotretinoin, is an anti-acne medication that works on the oil glands within the skin, shrinking them and diminishing their production.

6 common side effects include:
Dry eyes, mouth, lips, nose and skin
Itching
Nosebleeds
Muscle aches
Sun sensitivity
Poor night vision

21 serious side effects involve:
Depression and psychosis
Suicidal tendencies and attempts
Birth Defects
Ulcerative Colitis
Crohn's Disease
Inflammatory Bowel Disorder
Rectal Bleeding
Abdominal Pain
Premature Closure of Growth Plates

Desiccated Discs
Organ Damage
Optic Neuritis
Central Nervous System Injuries
Bone and Muscle Loss
Cardiovascular Injuries
Liver and Kidney Damage
Pancreatitis
Immune System Disorder
Lupus
Hearing and Vision Damage
Thyroid Disorders

Accutane is associated with severe birth defects, so it can't be taken safely by pregnant women or women who may become pregnant during the course of treatment. In fact, the drug carries such serious potential side-effects that women of reproductive age must participate in a Food and Drug Administration-approved monitoring program to receive a prescription for the drug.

In addition, the FDA has received over 100 reports of suicides linked to the use of Accutane, and over 1,000 reports of various psychological problems among those who use or have used the drug.

If you have taken Accutane and have experienced any unusual side effects, you should contact your physician at once. If you begin feeling depressed or suicidal, contact a psychiatric professional immediately. In addition, you can contact an attorney experienced in Accutane product liability litigation to discuss potential legal claims you might have, as you may be entitled to compensation for the damages Accutane has caused you.

The bottom line.

If you are willing to risk taking one of these medications for your acne, it is important to do so under the close supervision of your doctor to make sure that you can monitor the potential side effects.

If you're taking antibiotics or Accutane at the present time, you may want to consider stopping now. Also, if you have or are taking antibiotics, you will want to increase your consumption of probiotics such as yogurt, as this well help replenish your body's good bacteria and help rebuild your immune system.

If you are having any of the severe side effects mentioned above, you definitely want to stop taking these medications immediately. In most cases, your doctor will likely recommend tapering off these medications as soon as your symptoms begin to improve, or as soon as it becomes clear the drugs aren't helping — usually, within three to four months or less. Be sure to evaluate your options with your current health care provider.

Do your homework. Consult with a nutritionist to get the guidance you need to help you get rid of your acne naturally with lifestyle changes, stress reduction techniques, nutritional supplements, a proper diet and other natural treatments.

While there is no known cure for acne, it is treatable. And with proper treatment, acne will go away eventually, although not as quickly as any of us would like. Hang in there. Be patient. Be positive and your day will come.